KID-FRIENDLY RECIPES FOR TYPE 2 DIABETES

Fun & Delicious Meals for Managing Type 2 Diabetes in Children

T. John

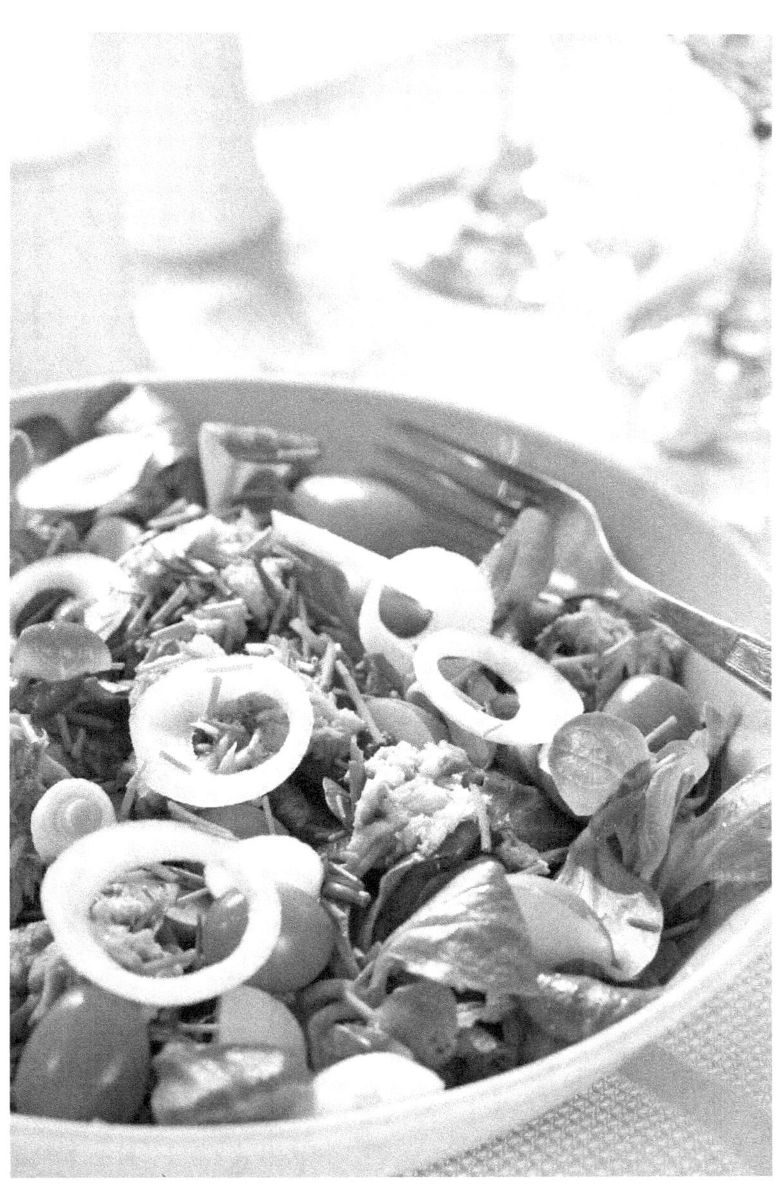

TABLE OF CONTENTS

Chapter 5: Snacks and Appetizers 100

Chapter 6: Desserts 117

INTRODUCTION

Imagine your child, a fearless explorer on the playground, suddenly diagnosed with a monster named type 2 diabetes. It can be scary, but with the right knowledge and a little creativity, you can turn this foe into a manageable friend. Let's break down this diabetes beast and craft a meal plan that's both delicious and keeps your little hero healthy.

Understanding the Sugar Gremlins:

Type 2 diabetes disrupts the body's ability to use sugar (glucose) for energy. Normally, sugar enters cells with the help of a hormone called insulin. In type 2 diabetes, either the body doesn't make enough insulin or the cells become resistant to it, leading to excess sugar in the bloodstream. This can cause tiredness, excessive thirst, and frequent urination.

The Superfood Squad: Healthy Eating Habits

Just like your child needs the right tools to conquer the jungle gym, they need the right foods to manage diabetes. Here's your healthy eating arsenal:

- **Veggie Power:** Fill half your child's plate with colorful vegetables like broccoli, carrots, and peppers. They're packed with vitamins, minerals, and fiber, keeping them energized without sugar spikes.

- **Whole-Grain Warriors:** Swap white bread, pasta, and rice for whole-wheat versions. These complex carbohydrates provide sustained energy and keep them feeling full for longer.

- **Lean Protein Protectors:** Include lean protein sources like grilled chicken, fish, or beans in every meal. Protein helps with growth and keeps blood sugar levels stable.

- **Healthy Fat Friends:** Don't ditch all fats! Healthy fats like avocado, nuts, and olive oil aid in nutrient absorption and keep your child feeling satisfied.

- **Limit Sugar Villains:** Sugary drinks, processed snacks, and candies are best enjoyed occasionally. They cause blood sugar spikes and can contribute to weight gain, making diabetes management harder.

Kid-Friendly Diabetic Recipe Rumble!

Here are some delicious recipes to get you started:

- **Breakfast Blitz:** Swap sugary cereals for a breakfast scramble with chopped veggies, whole-wheat toast soldiers for dipping, and a sprinkle of cheese.

- **Lunchtime Launch:** Pack a whole-wheat wrap filled with grilled chicken or tofu, lettuce, tomato, and a light yogurt dressing. Add some carrot sticks and baby bell peppers for a colorful crunch.

- **Snacktastic Adventure:** Instead of chips, try baked sweet potato fries with a sprinkle of cinnamon and a dollop of Greek yogurt for dipping. It's a sweet and satisfying alternative.

- **Dinner Dash:** Whip up a veggie-loaded stir-fry with lean protein like chicken or shrimp. Serve it over brown rice for a complete and flavorful meal.

- **Dessert Dazzle:** Bake muffins or cookies sweetened with applesauce or mashed banana instead of refined sugar. Top them with a dollop of low-fat yogurt for a guilt-free treat.

Remember:

- Get creative! Involve your child in the kitchen, letting them choose healthy ingredients and helping with age-appropriate tasks.
- Make it fun! Use cookie cutters to shape vegetables, have themed meals, or turn healthy eating into a game.

By working together, you can transform type 2 diabetes from a scary monster into a manageable foe. With a focus on healthy eating habits and delicious recipes, your child can be a thriving adventurer, diabetes or not!

Chapter 1: 30 Day Meal Plan

Week 1:

Day 1:

- Breakfast: Whole Grain Pancakes with Fresh Fruit Compote
- Lunch: Turkey and Veggie Wrap with Whole Wheat Tortilla
- Dinner: Baked Salmon with Roasted Vegetables
- Snack: Veggie Sticks with Hummus
- Dessert: Berry and Greek Yogurt Popsicles

Day 2:

- Breakfast: Veggie Egg Muffins
- Lunch: Chicken and Vegetable Stir-Fry with Brown Rice
- Dinner: Turkey Chili with Kidney Beans and Corn
- Snack: Apple Slices with Peanut Butter
- Dessert: Dark Chocolate-Dipped Strawberries

Day 3:

- Breakfast: Oatmeal Breakfast Bars
- Lunch: Tuna Salad Lettuce Wraps
- Dinner: Stuffed Bell Peppers with Lean Ground Beef and Quinoa
- Snack: Yogurt-Covered Frozen Grapes
- Dessert: Baked Apple Crisp with Oats and Cinnamon

Day 4:

- Breakfast: Greek Yogurt Parfait with Berries and Nuts
- Lunch: Mediterranean Quinoa Salad with Chickpeas and Feta
- Dinner: Veggie Stir-Fry with Tofu and Brown Rice
- Snack: Cheese and Whole Grain Crackers
- Dessert: Frozen Banana Bites with Dark Chocolate

Day 5:

- Breakfast: Breakfast Burrito with Lean Turkey and Veggies
- Lunch: Veggie and Hummus Sandwich on Multigrain Bread

- Dinner: Grilled Lemon Herb Chicken with Steamed Broccoli
- Snack: Popcorn with Parmesan Cheese
- Dessert: Lemon Blueberry Parfait with Granola

Day 6:

- Breakfast: Quinoa Breakfast Bowl with Spinach and Poached Egg
- Lunch: Turkey and Cheese Pinwheels with Spinach Wrap
- Dinner: Spaghetti Squash with Turkey Bolognese Sauce
- Snack: Trail Mix with Nuts and Dried Fruits
- Dessert: Chia Seed Pudding with Mixed Berries

Day 7:

- Breakfast: Banana Walnut Breakfast Cookies
- Lunch: Lentil Soup with Vegetables
- Dinner: BBQ Chicken Pizza with Whole Wheat Crust
- Snack: Cucumber and Tomato Salad with Balsamic Glaze

- Dessert: Pumpkin Pie Energy Bites

Week 2:

Day 8:

- Breakfast: Avocado Toast with Whole Grain Bread
- Lunch: Grilled Chicken Caesar Salad
- Dinner: Fish Tacos with Mango Salsa
- Snack: Edamame with Sea Salt
- Dessert: Greek Yogurt Bark with Berries and Nuts

Day 9:

- Breakfast: Berry Smoothie Bowl with Chia Seeds
- Lunch: Black Bean and Corn Quesadilla with Avocado
- Dinner: Turkey Meatballs with Zucchini Noodles
- Snack: Deviled Eggs with Greek Yogurt
- Dessert: Mango Sorbet with Lime Zest

Day 10:

- Breakfast: Apple Cinnamon Overnight Oats
- Lunch: Veggie Pasta Salad with Italian Dressing
- Dinner: Cauliflower Crust Veggie Pizza

- Snack: Guacamole with Baked Tortilla Chips
- Dessert: Almond Flour Chocolate Chip Cookies

Day 11:

- Breakfast: Sweet Potato Hash with Turkey Sausage
- Lunch: Turkey and Avocado Wrap with Whole Wheat Tortilla
- Dinner: Shrimp and Vegetable Skewers with Quinoa
- Snack: Carrot and Celery Sticks with Ranch Dip
- Dessert: Strawberry Banana Smoothie Bowl with Granola

Day 12:

- Breakfast: Spinach and Feta Crustless Quiche
- Lunch: Caprese Salad Skewers
- Dinner: Chicken and Broccoli Alfredo with Whole Wheat Pasta
- Snack: Greek Yogurt and Berry Popsicles
- Dessert: Coconut Macaroons with Dark Chocolate Drizzle

Day 13:

- Breakfast: Breakfast Quesadilla with Black Beans and Cheese
- Lunch: Chicken and Vegetable Kebabs with Quinoa
- Dinner: Beef and Vegetable Stir-Fry with Cauliflower Rice
- Snack: Whole Grain Pita Chips with Salsa
- Dessert: Frozen Yogurt Fruit Bark

Day 14:

- Breakfast: Mango Coconut Chia Pudding
- Lunch: Asian-inspired Broccoli and Beef Stir-Fry
- Dinner: Baked Sweet Potato with Black Bean Chili
- Snack: Cottage Cheese with Pineapple Chunks
- Dessert: Peanut Butter Banana Bites

Week 3:

Day 15:

- Breakfast: Peanut Butter Banana Smoothie
- Lunch: Greek Salad with Grilled Chicken
- Dinner: Grilled Veggie and Chicken Kabobs with Brown Rice

- Snack: Baked Sweet Potato Fries with Garlic Aioli
- Dessert: Avocado Chocolate Mousse

Day 16:

- Breakfast: Whole Grain Pancakes with Fresh Fruit Compote
- Lunch: Turkey and Veggie Wrap with Whole Wheat Tortilla
- Dinner: Baked Salmon with Roasted Vegetables
- Snack: Veggie Sticks with Hummus
- Dessert: Berry and Greek Yogurt Popsicles

Day 17:

- Breakfast: Veggie Egg Muffins
- Lunch: Chicken and Vegetable Stir-Fry with Brown Rice
- Dinner: Turkey Chili with Kidney Beans and Corn
- Snack: Apple Slices with Peanut Butter
- Dessert: Dark Chocolate-Dipped Strawberries

Day 18:

- Breakfast: Oatmeal Breakfast Bars

- Lunch: Tuna Salad Lettuce Wraps
- Dinner: Stuffed Bell Peppers with Lean Ground Beef and Quinoa
- Snack: Yogurt-Covered Frozen Grapes
- Dessert: Baked Apple Crisp with Oats and Cinnamon

Day 19:

- Breakfast: Greek Yogurt Parfait with Berries and Nuts
- Lunch: Mediterranean Quinoa Salad with Chickpeas and Feta
- Dinner: Veggie Stir-Fry with Tofu and Brown Rice
- Snack: Cheese and Whole Grain Crackers
- Dessert: Frozen Banana Bites with Dark Chocolate

Day 20:

- Breakfast: Breakfast Burrito with Lean Turkey and Veggies
- Lunch: Veggie and Hummus Sandwich on Multigrain Bread
- Dinner: Grilled Lemon Herb Chicken with Steamed Broccoli

- Snack: Popcorn with Parmesan Cheese
- Dessert: Lemon Blueberry Parfait with Granola

Day 21:

- Breakfast: Quinoa Breakfast Bowl with Spinach and Poached Egg
- Lunch: Turkey and Cheese Pinwheels with Spinach Wrap
- Dinner: Spaghetti Squash with Turkey Bolognese Sauce
- Snack: Trail Mix with Nuts and Dried Fruits
- Dessert: Chia Seed Pudding with Mixed Berries

Week 4:

Day 22:

- Breakfast: Banana Walnut Breakfast Cookies
- Lunch: Lentil Soup with Vegetables
- Dinner: BBQ Chicken Pizza with Whole Wheat Crust
- Snack: Cucumber and Tomato Salad with Balsamic Glaze
- Dessert: Pumpkin Pie Energy Bites

Day 23:

- Breakfast: Avocado Toast with Whole Grain Bread
- Lunch: Grilled Chicken Caesar Salad
- Dinner: Fish Tacos with Mango Salsa
- Snack: Edamame with Sea Salt
- Dessert: Greek Yogurt Bark with Berries and Nuts

Day 24:

- Breakfast: Berry Smoothie Bowl with Chia Seeds
- Lunch: Black Bean and Corn Quesadilla with Avocado
- Dinner: Turkey Meatballs with Zucchini Noodles
- Snack: Deviled Eggs with Greek Yogurt
- Dessert: Mango Sorbet with Lime Zest

Day 25:

- Breakfast: Apple Cinnamon Overnight Oats
- Lunch: Veggie Pasta Salad with Italian Dressing
- Dinner: Cauliflower Crust Veggie Pizza
- Snack: Guacamole with Baked Tortilla Chips
- Dessert: Almond Flour Chocolate Chip Cookies

Day 26:

- Breakfast: Sweet Potato Hash with Turkey Sausage
- Lunch: Turkey and Avocado Wrap with Whole Wheat Tortilla
- Dinner: Shrimp and Vegetable Skewers with Quinoa
- Snack: Carrot and Celery Sticks with Ranch Dip
- Dessert: Strawberry Banana Smoothie Bowl with Granola

Day 27:

- Breakfast: Spinach and Feta Crustless Quiche
- Lunch: Caprese Salad Skewers
- Dinner: Chicken and Broccoli Alfredo with Whole Wheat Pasta
- Snack: Greek Yogurt and Berry Popsicles
- Dessert: Coconut Macaroons with Dark Chocolate Drizzle

Day 28:

- Breakfast: Breakfast Quesadilla with Black Beans and Cheese
- Lunch: Chicken and Vegetable Kebabs with Quinoa

- Dinner: Beef and Vegetable Stir-Fry with Cauliflower Rice
- Snack: Whole Grain Pita Chips with Salsa
- Dessert: Frozen Yogurt Fruit Bark

Day 29:

- Breakfast: Mango Coconut Chia Pudding
- Lunch: Asian-inspired Broccoli and Beef Stir-Fry
- Dinner: Baked Sweet Potato with Black Bean Chili
- Snack: Cottage Cheese with Pineapple Chunks
- Dessert: Peanut Butter Banana Bites

Day 30:

- Breakfast: Peanut Butter Banana Smoothie
- Lunch: Greek Salad with Grilled Chicken
- Dinner: Grilled Veggie and Chicken Kabobs with Brown Rice
- Snack: Baked Sweet Potato Fries with Garlic Aioli
- Dessert: Avocado Chocolate Mousse

Chapter 2: Breakfast Recipes

In this chapter, we present delicious and kid-friendly breakfast recipes that are not only packed with flavor but also designed to support a balanced diet for children with type 2 diabetes. From hearty pancakes to refreshing smoothie bowls, these recipes incorporate wholesome ingredients to ensure a satisfying and nutritious start to the morning.

Whole Grain Pancakes with Fresh Fruit Compote

Ingredients:

- 1 cup whole wheat flour
- 1 tablespoon baking powder
- 1 tablespoon honey
- 1 cup low-fat milk
- 1 egg
- 1 teaspoon vanilla extract
- Fresh mixed fruit (e.g., berries, sliced bananas)
- 1 tablespoon maple syrup (optional)

Instructions:

1. In a mixing bowl, combine whole wheat flour and baking powder.
2. In a separate bowl, whisk together honey, low-fat milk, egg, and vanilla extract.
3. Gradually add the wet ingredients to the dry ingredients, stirring until just combined.
4. Heat a non-stick skillet over medium heat and lightly coat with cooking spray.
5. Pour 1/4 cup of batter onto the skillet for each pancake.
6. Cook until bubbles form on the surface, then flip and cook until golden brown.
7. Serve pancakes topped with fresh fruit compote and a drizzle of maple syrup, if desired.

Nutrition Information:

- Calories: 250
- Protein: 8g
- Carbohydrates: 45g
- Fat: 4g
- Fiber: 6g

- Sugar: 12g
- Portion Size: 2 pancakes

Veggie Egg Muffins

Ingredients:

- 6 eggs
- 1/4 cup diced bell peppers
- 1/4 cup diced onions
- 1/4 cup chopped spinach
- Salt and pepper to taste
- Cooking spray

Instructions:

1. Preheat the oven to 350°F (175°C) and lightly grease a muffin tin with cooking spray.
2. In a mixing bowl, whisk together eggs, bell peppers, onions, spinach, salt, and pepper.
3. Pour the egg mixture evenly into the muffin cups, filling each about 3/4 full.
4. Bake for 20-25 minutes or until the egg muffins are set and lightly golden on top.

5. Allow to cool slightly before removing from the muffin tin.

6. Serve warm or store in the refrigerator for quick breakfast options throughout the week.

Nutrition Information:

- Calories: 80
- Protein: 6g
- Carbohydrates: 2g
- Fat: 5g
- Fiber: 0.5g
- Sugar: 1g
- Portion Size: 2 egg muffins

Oatmeal Breakfast Bars

Ingredients:

- 2 cups rolled oats
- 1/2 cup almond butter
- 1/4 cup honey
- 1/4 cup unsweetened applesauce
- 1/4 cup dried cranberries
- 1/4 cup chopped nuts (e.g., almonds, walnuts)

- 1 teaspoon cinnamon
- Pinch of salt

Instructions:

1. Preheat the oven to 350°F (175°C) and line a baking dish with parchment paper.
2. In a large mixing bowl, combine rolled oats, almond butter, honey, applesauce, dried cranberries, chopped nuts, cinnamon, and salt.
3. Mix until all ingredients are well combined and the mixture sticks together.
4. Press the mixture evenly into the prepared baking dish.
5. Bake for 20-25 minutes or until the edges are golden brown.
6. Allow to cool completely before cutting into bars.
7. Store in an airtight container for up to one week.

Nutrition Information:

- Calories: 180
- Protein: 5g
- Carbohydrates: 20g

- Fat: 9g
- Fiber: 3g
- Sugar: 8g
- Portion Size: 1 bar

Greek Yogurt Parfait with Berries and Nuts

Ingredients:

- 1 cup low-fat Greek yogurt
- 1/4 cup mixed berries (e.g., strawberries, blueberries, raspberries)
- 2 tablespoons chopped nuts (e.g., almonds, walnuts)
- 1 tablespoon honey (optional)

Instructions:

1. In a serving glass or bowl, layer Greek yogurt, mixed berries, and chopped nuts.
2. Drizzle with honey if desired for added sweetness.
3. Repeat layers until ingredients are used up.
4. Serve immediately or refrigerate for later.

Nutrition Information:

- Calories: 200
- Protein: 15g
- Carbohydrates: 20g
- Fat: 7g
- Fiber: 3g
- Sugar: 15g
- Portion Size: 1 parfait

Breakfast Burrito with Lean Turkey and Veggies

Ingredients:

- 2 large whole wheat tortillas
- 4 eggs
- 1/2 cup diced bell peppers
- 1/4 cup diced onions
- 1/4 cup diced tomatoes
- 1/4 cup cooked lean ground turkey
- Salt and pepper to taste
- Salsa or hot sauce for serving (optional)

Instructions:

1. In a skillet, scramble the eggs over medium heat until cooked through.
2. Remove the eggs from the skillet and set aside.
3. In the same skillet, sauté diced bell peppers, onions, and tomatoes until softened.
4. Add cooked lean ground turkey to the skillet and cook until heated through.
5. Season with salt and pepper to taste.
6. Warm the whole wheat tortillas in the microwave or on a skillet.
7. Divide the scrambled eggs and turkey-vegetable mixture evenly between the tortillas.
8. Roll up the tortillas to form burritos.
9. Serve with salsa or hot sauce if desired.

Nutrition Information:

- Calories: 300
- Protein: 20g
- Carbohydrates: 30g
- Fat: 10g
- Fiber: 6g

- Sugar: 3g
- Portion Size: 1 burrito

Quinoa Breakfast Bowl with Spinach and Poached Egg

Ingredients:

- 1/2 cup cooked quinoa
- 1 cup fresh spinach leaves
- 1 poached egg
- Salt and pepper to taste
- Optional toppings: sliced avocado, cherry tomatoes, hot sauce

Instructions:

1. In a serving bowl, layer cooked quinoa and fresh spinach leaves.
2. Top with a poached egg and season with salt and pepper.
3. Add optional toppings such as sliced avocado, cherry tomatoes, or hot sauce if desired.
4. Serve immediately.

Nutrition Information:

- Calories: 250
- Protein: 15g
- Carbohydrates: 25g
- Fat: 10g
- Fiber: 6g
- Sugar: 1g
- Portion Size: 1 bowl

Banana Walnut Breakfast Cookies

Ingredients:

- 2 ripe bananas, mashed
- 1 cup rolled oats
- 1/4 cup chopped walnuts
- 1 tablespoon honey
- 1/2 teaspoon cinnamon
- Pinch of salt

Instructions:

1. Preheat the oven to 350°F (175°C) and line a baking sheet with parchment paper.

2. In a mixing bowl, combine mashed bananas, rolled oats, chopped walnuts, honey, cinnamon, and salt.

3. Mix until all ingredients are well combined.

4. Drop spoonfuls of the mixture onto the prepared baking sheet, forming cookies.

5. Bake for 12-15 minutes or until the cookies are golden brown.

6. Allow to cool on the baking sheet for a few minutes before transferring to a wire rack to cool completely.

7. Enjoy as a grab-and-go breakfast or snack.

Nutrition Information:

- Calories: 90
- Protein: 2g
- Carbohydrates: 15g
- Fat: 3g
- Fiber: 2g
- Sugar: 6g
- Portion Size: 2 cookies

Avocado Toast with Whole Grain Bread

Ingredients:

- 2 slices whole grain bread, toasted
- 1 ripe avocado
- Salt and pepper to taste
- Optional toppings: sliced tomatoes, red pepper flakes, sesame seeds

Instructions:

1. Toast the whole grain bread slices until golden brown.
2. In a small bowl, mash the ripe avocado with a fork until smooth.
3. Season with salt and pepper to taste.
4. Spread the mashed avocado evenly onto the toasted bread slices.
5. Top with optional toppings such as sliced tomatoes, red pepper flakes, or sesame seeds if desired.
6. Serve immediately.

Nutrition Information:

- Calories: 200
- Protein: 5g
- Carbohydrates: 20g
- Fat: 12g
- Fiber: 7g
- Sugar: 2g
- Portion Size: 1 avocado toast

Berry Smoothie Bowl with Chia Seeds

Ingredients:

- 1 cup mixed berries (e.g., strawberries, blueberries, raspberries)
- 1/2 frozen banana
- 1/2 cup low-fat Greek yogurt
- 1 tablespoon chia seeds
- 1/4 cup almond milk
- Optional toppings: sliced almonds, shredded coconut, granola

Instructions:

1. In a blender, combine mixed berries, frozen banana, Greek yogurt, chia seeds, and almond milk.
2. Blend until smooth and creamy, adding more almond milk if needed to reach desired consistency.
3. Pour the smoothie into a bowl.
4. Top with sliced almonds, shredded coconut, and granola for added texture and flavor.
5. Serve immediately with a spoon.

Nutrition Information:

- Calories: 250
- Protein: 12g
- Carbohydrates: 30g
- Fat: 10g
- Fiber: 8g
- Sugar: 16g
- Portion Size: 1 smoothie bowl

Apple Cinnamon Overnight Oats

Ingredients:

- 1/2 cup rolled oats

- 1/2 cup low-fat milk or almond milk
- 1/2 cup unsweetened applesauce
- 1 tablespoon honey
- 1/2 teaspoon cinnamon
- 1/4 cup diced apples
- Optional toppings: sliced almonds, raisins, cinnamon

Instructions:

1. In a mason jar or container, combine rolled oats, milk, applesauce, honey, and cinnamon.
2. Stir in diced apples until well combined.
3. Cover and refrigerate overnight or for at least 4 hours.
4. Before serving, stir the overnight oats and top with optional toppings such as sliced almonds, raisins, or additional cinnamon.
5. Enjoy cold or warm by heating in the microwave for 1-2 minutes.

Nutrition Information:

- Calories: 280
- Protein: 8g

- Carbohydrates: 50g

- Fat: 6g

- Fiber: 7g

- Sugar: 20g

- Portion Size: 1 serving

Sweet Potato Hash with Turkey Sausage

Ingredients:

- 2 medium sweet potatoes, peeled and diced

- 1/2 lb lean turkey sausage, casings removed

- 1/2 onion, diced

- 1 bell pepper, diced

- 2 cloves garlic, minced

- Salt and pepper to taste

- 1 tablespoon olive oil

Instructions:

1. In a large skillet, heat olive oil over medium heat.

2. Add diced sweet potatoes and cook until slightly tender, about 5-7 minutes.

3. Add lean turkey sausage, breaking it up with a spatula, and cook until browned.

4. Stir in diced onion, bell pepper, and minced garlic. Cook until vegetables are softened.

5. Season with salt and pepper to taste.

6. Serve hot as a hearty breakfast option.

Nutrition Information:

- Calories: 280
- Protein: 15g
- Carbohydrates: 25g
- Fat: 12g
- Fiber: 4g
- Sugar: 7g
- Portion Size: 1 cup

Spinach and Feta Crustless Quiche

Ingredients:

- 6 eggs
- 1 cup low-fat milk
- 2 cups fresh spinach leaves
- 1/2 cup crumbled feta cheese

- Salt and pepper to taste
- Cooking spray

Instructions:

1. Preheat the oven to 350°F (175°C) and lightly grease a pie dish with cooking spray.
2. In a mixing bowl, whisk together eggs and low-fat milk.
3. Stir in fresh spinach leaves and crumbled feta cheese.
4. Season with salt and pepper to taste.
5. Pour the egg mixture into the prepared pie dish.
6. Bake for 25-30 minutes or until the quiche is set and lightly golden on top.
7. Allow to cool slightly before slicing and serving.

Nutrition Information:

- Calories: 180
- Protein: 12g
- Carbohydrates: 5g
- Fat: 10g
- Fiber: 1g
- Sugar: 3g
- Portion Size: 1 slice

Breakfast Quesadilla with Black Beans and Cheese

Ingredients:

- 2 whole wheat tortillas
- 1/2 cup black beans, drained and rinsed
- 1/2 cup shredded low-fat cheese
- 2 eggs, scrambled
- 1/4 cup salsa
- Cooking spray

Instructions:

1. Heat a non-stick skillet over medium heat and lightly coat with cooking spray.
2. Place one whole wheat tortilla in the skillet and sprinkle half of the shredded cheese evenly over the tortilla.
3. Spread scrambled eggs and black beans over the cheese.
4. Top with the remaining shredded cheese and place the second tortilla on top.
5. Cook for 2-3 minutes on each side or until the quesadilla is golden brown and the cheese is melted.
6. Slice into wedges and serve with salsa on the side.

Nutrition Information:

- Calories: 350
- Protein: 20g
- Carbohydrates: 30g
- Fat: 15g
- Fiber: 8g
- Sugar: 2g
- Portion Size: 1 quesadilla

Mango Coconut Chia Pudding

Ingredients:

- 1/4 cup chia seeds
- 1 cup unsweetened coconut milk
- 1/2 cup diced mango
- 1 tablespoon honey or maple syrup (optional)
- Shredded coconut for garnish (optional)

Instructions:

1. In a bowl, combine chia seeds and coconut milk. Stir well to combine.

2. Cover and refrigerate for at least 2 hours or overnight, allowing the chia seeds to absorb the liquid and thicken.

3. Before serving, stir in diced mango and honey or maple syrup if desired.

4. Divide the chia pudding into serving bowls and garnish with shredded coconut if desired.

5. Serve chilled as a refreshing breakfast option.

Nutrition Information:

- Calories: 220
- Protein: 5g
- Carbohydrates: 25g
- Fat: 12g
- Fiber: 10g
- Sugar: 10g
- Portion Size: 1 serving

Peanut Butter Banana Smoothie

Ingredients:

- 1 ripe banana
- 2 tablespoons natural peanut butter

- 1 cup low-fat milk or almond milk
- 1/2 cup plain Greek yogurt
- 1 tablespoon honey or maple syrup (optional)
- Ice cubes (optional)

Instructions:

1. In a blender, combine ripe banana, natural peanut butter, low-fat milk or almond milk, and plain Greek yogurt.
2. Add honey or maple syrup if additional sweetness is desired.
3. Optional: Add ice cubes for a colder and thicker consistency.
4. Blend until smooth and creamy.
5. Pour into glasses and serve immediately.

Nutrition Information:

- Calories: 300
- Protein: 15g
- Carbohydrates: 30g
- Fat: 15g
- Fiber: 3g
- Sugar: 20g
- Portion Size: 1 smoothie

Chapter 3: Lunch Recipes

These recipes are crafted with wholesome ingredients and balanced nutrition to keep energy levels stable throughout the day while supporting overall health. From wraps to salads to hearty soups, each dish offers a burst of flavors and textures that will satisfy your taste buds without compromising your wellness goals.

Turkey and Veggie Wrap with Whole Wheat Tortilla

Ingredients:

- 4 ounces sliced turkey breast
- 1 whole wheat tortilla
- 1/4 cup shredded lettuce
- 1/4 cup sliced cucumbers
- 1/4 cup shredded carrots
- 2 tablespoons hummus
- Salt and pepper to taste

Instructions:

1. Lay the whole wheat tortilla flat on a clean surface.

2. Spread hummus evenly over the tortilla.

3. Layer the turkey slices, shredded lettuce, cucumbers, and shredded carrots on top of the hummus.

4. Season with salt and pepper to taste.

5. Roll the tortilla tightly, folding in the sides as you go.

6. Slice the wrap in half diagonally.

7. Serve and enjoy!

Nutrition Information (per serving):

- Calories: 280
- Protein: 20g
- Carbohydrates: 30g
- Fat: 8g
- Fiber: 6g
- Sugar: 4g
- Portion Size: 1 wrap

Chicken and Vegetable Stir-Fry with Brown Rice

Ingredients:

- 1 tablespoon olive oil
- 8 ounces boneless, skinless chicken breast, sliced
- 2 cups mixed vegetables (such as bell peppers, broccoli, and snap peas)
- 2 cloves garlic, minced
- 1/4 cup low-sodium soy sauce
- 2 cups cooked brown rice

Instructions:

1. Heat olive oil in a large skillet over medium heat.
2. Add sliced chicken breast to the skillet and cook until browned and cooked through.
3. Add mixed vegetables and minced garlic to the skillet, and stir-fry until vegetables are tender-crisp.
4. Pour soy sauce over the chicken and vegetable mixture, and stir to coat evenly.
5. Serve the stir-fry over cooked brown rice.
6. Enjoy!

Nutrition Information (per serving):

- Calories: 320

- Protein: 25g

- Carbohydrates: 35g

- Fat: 9g

- Fiber: 6g

- Sugar: 3g

- Portion Size: 1 cup stir-fry with 1/2 cup brown rice

Tuna Salad Lettuce Wraps

Ingredients:

- 1 can (5 ounces) tuna, drained

- 2 tablespoons Greek yogurt

- 1 tablespoon Dijon mustard

- 1/4 cup diced celery

- 1/4 cup diced red onion

- Salt and pepper to taste

- 4 large lettuce leaves

Instructions:

1. In a bowl, combine drained tuna, Greek yogurt, Dijon mustard, diced celery, and diced red onion.

2. Mix well until all ingredients are evenly incorporated.

3. Season with salt and pepper to taste.

4. Divide the tuna salad mixture evenly among the lettuce leaves.

5. Roll up the lettuce leaves to form wraps.

6. Serve and enjoy!

Nutrition Information (per serving):

- Calories: 120
- Protein: 15g
- Carbohydrates: 5g
- Fat: 5g
- Fiber: 1g
- Sugar: 2g
- Portion Size: 1 lettuce wrap

Mediterranean Quinoa Salad with Chickpeas and Feta

Ingredients:

- 1 cup cooked quinoa

- 1 can (15 ounces) chickpeas, drained and rinsed
- 1/2 cup diced cucumber
- 1/2 cup halved cherry tomatoes
- 1/4 cup chopped Kalamata olives
- 2 tablespoons crumbled feta cheese
- 2 tablespoons chopped fresh parsley
- 2 tablespoons extra virgin olive oil
- 1 tablespoon lemon juice
- Salt and pepper to taste

Instructions:

1. In a large bowl, combine cooked quinoa, chickpeas, diced cucumber, halved cherry tomatoes, chopped Kalamata olives, crumbled feta cheese, and chopped fresh parsley.
2. Drizzle extra virgin olive oil and lemon juice over the salad.
3. Season with salt and pepper to taste.
4. Toss the salad until all ingredients are well combined.
5. Serve chilled or at room temperature.
6. Enjoy!

Nutrition Information (per serving):

- Calories: 280
- Protein: 10g
- Carbohydrates: 30g
- Fat: 12g
- Fiber: 6g
- Sugar: 3g
- Portion Size: 1 cup salad

Veggie and Hummus Sandwich on Multigrain Bread

Ingredients:

- 2 slices multigrain bread
- 2 tablespoons hummus
- 1/4 cup sliced cucumbers
- 1/4 cup sliced bell peppers
- 1/4 cup shredded carrots
- 1/4 cup baby spinach leaves

Instructions:

1. Spread hummus evenly on one side of each slice of multigrain bread.
2. Layer sliced cucumbers, bell peppers, shredded carrots, and baby spinach leaves on one slice of bread.
3. Place the other slice of bread on top to form a sandwich.
4. Slice the sandwich in half diagonally.
5. Serve and enjoy!

Nutrition Information (per serving):

- Calories: 250
- Protein: 8g
- Carbohydrates: 40g
- Fat: 6g
- Fiber: 8g
- Sugar: 6g
- Portion Size: 1 sandwich

Turkey and Cheese Pinwheels with Spinach Wrap

Ingredients:

- 2 large spinach wraps
- 4 slices turkey breast
- 2 slices low-fat cheese
- 1/4 cup baby spinach leaves
- 2 tablespoons mustard or mayonnaise (optional)

Instructions:

1. Lay the spinach wraps flat on a clean surface.
2. Spread mustard or mayonnaise (if using) evenly over each wrap.
3. Layer two slices of turkey breast and one slice of low-fat cheese on each wrap.
4. Place baby spinach leaves on top of the turkey and cheese.
5. Roll up the wraps tightly to form pinwheels.
6. Slice the pinwheels into bite-sized pieces.
7. Serve and enjoy!

Nutrition Information (per serving):

- Calories: 180
- Protein: 15g
- Carbohydrates: 15g
- Fat: 7g
- Fiber: 2g
- Sugar: 1g
- Portion Size: 2 pinwheels

Lentil Soup with Vegetables

Ingredients:

- 1 cup dried green lentils, rinsed and drained
- 4 cups low-sodium vegetable broth
- 1 onion, chopped
- 2 carrots, diced
- 2 celery stalks, diced
- 2 cloves garlic, minced
- 1 teaspoon ground cumin
- 1 teaspoon ground coriander
- Salt and pepper to taste
- Fresh parsley for garnish (optional)

Instructions:

1. In a large pot, combine dried green lentils, low-sodium vegetable broth, chopped onion, diced carrots, diced celery, minced garlic, ground cumin, and ground coriander.
2. Bring the mixture to a boil over medium-high heat.
3. Reduce heat to low, cover, and simmer for 25-30 minutes, or until lentils and vegetables are tender.
4. Season with salt and pepper to taste.
5. Ladle the soup into bowls and garnish with fresh parsley if desired.
6. Serve hot and enjoy!

Nutrition Information (per serving):

- Calories: 220
- Protein: 15g
- Carbohydrates: 35g
- Fat: 1g
- Fiber: 15g
- Sugar: 5g
- Portion Size: 1 cup soup

Grilled Chicken Caesar Salad

Ingredients:

- 8 ounces grilled chicken breast, sliced
- 4 cups chopped romaine lettuce
- 1/4 cup grated Parmesan cheese
- 1/4 cup whole wheat croutons
- 2 tablespoons Caesar dressing (look for a low-sugar option)

Instructions:

1. In a large bowl, combine chopped romaine lettuce, grilled chicken breast slices, grated Parmesan cheese, and whole wheat croutons.
2. Drizzle Caesar dressing over the salad.
3. Toss the salad until all ingredients are well coated with dressing.
4. Divide the salad into individual serving bowls.
5. Serve immediately and enjoy!

Nutrition Information (per serving):

- Calories: 280
- Protein: 30g

- Carbohydrates: 10g

- Fat: 12g

- Fiber: 3g

- Sugar: 2g

- Portion Size: 2 cups salad

Black Bean and Corn Quesadilla with Avocado

Ingredients:

- 1 whole wheat tortilla

- 1/4 cup canned black beans, drained and rinsed

- 1/4 cup frozen corn, thawed

- 1/4 cup shredded cheddar cheese

- 1/4 avocado, sliced

- Salsa and Greek yogurt for serving (optional)

Instructions:

1. Heat a non-stick skillet over medium heat.

2. Place the whole wheat tortilla in the skillet and warm it for about 1 minute on each side.

3. Remove the tortilla from the skillet and set it aside.

4. On one half of the tortilla, spread black beans, thawed corn, shredded cheddar cheese, and sliced avocado.

5. Fold the other half of the tortilla over the filling to form a half-moon shape.

6. Return the quesadilla to the skillet and cook for 2-3 minutes on each side, or until cheese is melted and tortilla is crispy.

7. Remove from the skillet, slice into wedges, and serve with salsa and Greek yogurt if desired.

Nutrition Information (per serving):

- Calories: 320
- Protein: 15g
- Carbohydrates: 35g
- Fat: 14g
- Fiber: 9g
- Sugar: 2g
- Portion Size: 1 quesadilla

Veggie Pasta Salad with Italian Dressing

Ingredients:

- 2 cups cooked whole wheat pasta
- 1 cup cherry tomatoes, halved
- 1/2 cup diced bell peppers (any color)
- 1/2 cup diced cucumber
- 1/4 cup sliced black olives
- 1/4 cup diced red onion
- 2 tablespoons chopped fresh basil
- 2 tablespoons chopped fresh parsley
- 1/4 cup Italian dressing (look for a low-sugar option)

Instructions:

1. In a large bowl, combine cooked whole wheat pasta, cherry tomatoes, diced bell peppers, diced cucumber, sliced black olives, diced red onion, chopped fresh basil, and chopped fresh parsley.
2. Drizzle Italian dressing over the pasta salad.
3. Toss the salad until all ingredients are well coated with dressing.

4. Chill in the refrigerator for at least 30 minutes before serving to allow the flavors to meld.

5. Serve cold and enjoy!

Nutrition Information (per serving):

- Calories: 250
- Protein: 8g
- Carbohydrates: 35g
- Fat: 8g
- Fiber: 6g
- Sugar: 4g
- Portion Size: 1 cup salad

Turkey and Avocado Wrap with Whole Wheat Tortilla

Ingredients:

- 1 whole wheat tortilla
- 3 ounces sliced turkey breast
- 1/4 avocado, sliced
- 1/4 cup shredded lettuce
- 1/4 cup diced tomatoes

- 1 tablespoon Greek yogurt (optional)
- Salt and pepper to taste

Instructions:

1. Lay the whole wheat tortilla flat on a clean surface.
2. Layer sliced turkey breast, sliced avocado, shredded lettuce, and diced tomatoes on top of the tortilla.
3. Optionally, spread Greek yogurt evenly over the ingredients.
4. Season with salt and pepper to taste.
5. Roll up the tortilla tightly, folding in the sides as you go.
6. Slice the wrap in half diagonally.
7. Serve and enjoy!

Nutrition Information (per serving):

- Calories: 280
- Protein: 20g
- Carbohydrates: 25g
- Fat: 10g
- Fiber: 6g
- Sugar: 2g

- Portion Size: 1 wrap

Caprese Salad Skewers

Ingredients:

- 12 cherry tomatoes
- 12 fresh mozzarella balls (bocconcini)
- 12 fresh basil leaves
- 1 tablespoon balsamic glaze
- Salt and pepper to taste
- Wooden skewers

Instructions:

1. Thread a cherry tomato, a fresh mozzarella ball, and a fresh basil leaf onto each wooden skewer, repeating until all ingredients are used.
2. Arrange the skewers on a serving platter.
3. Drizzle balsamic glaze over the skewers.
4. Season with salt and pepper to taste.
5. Serve as an appetizer or side dish.
6. Enjoy!

Nutrition Information (per serving, 3 skewers):

- Calories: 120
- Protein: 8g
- Carbohydrates: 4g
- Fat: 8g
- Fiber: 1g
- Sugar: 2g
- Portion Size: 3 skewers

Chicken and Vegetable Kebabs with Quinoa

Ingredients:

- 8 ounces boneless, skinless chicken breast, cut into cubes
- 1 bell pepper, cut into chunks
- 1 zucchini, sliced
- 1 onion, cut into wedges
- 1 cup cooked quinoa
- 2 tablespoons olive oil
- 1 teaspoon Italian seasoning
- Salt and pepper to taste

- Wooden skewers

Instructions:

1. In a bowl, combine cubed chicken breast, bell pepper chunks, sliced zucchini, onion wedges, olive oil, Italian seasoning, salt, and pepper. Toss until well coated.
2. Thread the marinated chicken and vegetables onto wooden skewers, alternating between chicken and vegetables.
3. Preheat a grill or grill pan over medium-high heat.
4. Grill the kebabs for 8-10 minutes, turning occasionally, until the chicken is cooked through and the vegetables are tender.
5. Serve the kebabs over cooked quinoa.
6. Enjoy!

Nutrition Information (per serving):

- Calories: 320
- Protein: 25g
- Carbohydrates: 20g
- Fat: 15g

- Fiber: 3g

- Sugar: 3g

- Portion Size: 2 kebabs with 1/2 cup quinoa

Asian-inspired Broccoli and Beef Stir-Fry

Ingredients:

- 8 ounces flank steak, thinly sliced

- 2 cups broccoli florets

- 1 bell pepper, sliced

- 1 carrot, julienned

- 2 cloves garlic, minced

- 2 tablespoons low-sodium soy sauce

- 1 tablespoon hoisin sauce

- 1 tablespoon sesame oil

- 1 teaspoon cornstarch

- 2 green onions, sliced (for garnish)

- Cooked brown rice for serving

Instructions:

1. In a small bowl, whisk together soy sauce, hoisin sauce, sesame oil, and cornstarch to make the sauce.
2. Heat a large skillet or wok over high heat.
3. Add thinly sliced flank steak to the skillet and cook until browned on all sides, about 2-3 minutes. Remove from skillet and set aside.
4. In the same skillet, add broccoli florets, sliced bell pepper, julienned carrot, and minced garlic. Stir-fry for 3-4 minutes, or until vegetables are tender-crisp.
5. Return the cooked flank steak to the skillet.
6. Pour the prepared sauce over the beef and vegetables, stirring well to coat everything evenly.
7. Cook for an additional 1-2 minutes, or until the sauce has thickened slightly.
8. Remove from heat and garnish with sliced green onions.
9. Serve the stir-fry hot over cooked brown rice.
10. Enjoy!

Nutrition Information (per serving):

- Calories: 320

- Protein: 25g
- Carbohydrates: 20g
- Fat: 15g
- Fiber: 4g
- Sugar: 6g
- Portion Size: 1 cup stir-fry with 1/2 cup brown rice

Greek Salad with Grilled Chicken

Ingredients:

- 8 ounces grilled chicken breast, sliced
- 4 cups chopped romaine lettuce
- 1/2 cucumber, sliced
- 1/2 cup cherry tomatoes, halved
- 1/4 cup sliced red onion
- 1/4 cup sliced Kalamata olives
- 1/4 cup crumbled feta cheese
- 2 tablespoons extra virgin olive oil
- 1 tablespoon red wine vinegar
- 1 teaspoon dried oregano
- Salt and pepper to taste

Instructions:

1. In a large bowl, combine chopped romaine lettuce, sliced cucumber, halved cherry tomatoes, sliced red onion, sliced Kalamata olives, and crumbled feta cheese.
2. In a small bowl, whisk together extra virgin olive oil, red wine vinegar, dried oregano, salt, and pepper to make the dressing.
3. Drizzle the dressing over the salad and toss until well coated.
4. Divide the salad into individual serving bowls.
5. Top each serving with sliced grilled chicken breast.
6. Serve immediately and enjoy!

Nutrition Information (per serving):

- Calories: 280
- Protein: 25g
- Carbohydrates: 10g
- Fat: 15g
- Fiber: 3g
- Sugar: 4g

- Portion Size: 2 cups salad with 4 ounces grilled chicken

Chapter 4: Dinner Recipes

These recipes are carefully crafted to be both delicious and suitable for individuals managing type 2 diabetes. From succulent salmon to flavorful stir-fries, each dish offers a balance of protein, vegetables, and whole grains to support overall well-being. Let's explore these nutritious and satisfying dinner options below.

Baked Salmon with Roasted Vegetables

Ingredients:

- 4 salmon fillets
- 2 cups mixed vegetables (such as bell peppers, zucchini, and cherry tomatoes)
- 2 tablespoons olive oil
- Salt and pepper to taste
- Lemon wedges for serving

Instructions:

1. Preheat the oven to 400°F (200°C).

2. Place the salmon fillets on a baking sheet lined with parchment paper.

3. Arrange the mixed vegetables around the salmon.

4. Drizzle olive oil over the salmon and vegetables, then season with salt and pepper.

5. Bake for 15-20 minutes, or until the salmon is cooked through and the vegetables are tender.

6. Serve hot with lemon wedges on the side.

Nutrition Information:

- Calories: 350
- Protein: 25g
- Carbohydrates: 10g
- Fat: 22g
- Fiber: 3g
- Sugar: 5g
- Portion Size: 1 fillet with vegetables

Turkey Chili with Kidney Beans and Corn

Ingredients:

- 1 lb ground turkey
- 1 onion, diced
- 2 cloves garlic, minced
- 1 can (15 oz) kidney beans, drained and rinsed
- 1 can (15 oz) corn kernels, drained
- 1 can (15 oz) diced tomatoes
- 1 cup chicken broth
- 2 tablespoons chili powder
- 1 teaspoon cumin
- Salt and pepper to taste
- Optional toppings: shredded cheese, Greek yogurt, sliced green onions

Instructions:

1. In a large pot, cook ground turkey over medium heat until browned.
2. Add diced onion and minced garlic, cooking until softened.

3. Stir in kidney beans, corn, diced tomatoes, chicken broth, chili powder, cumin, salt, and pepper.

4. Bring the chili to a simmer and let it cook for 20-25 minutes, stirring occasionally.

5. Serve hot, topped with optional toppings if desired.

Nutrition Information:

- Calories: 300
- Protein: 22g
- Carbohydrates: 30g
- Fat: 10g
- Fiber: 8g
- Sugar: 6g
- Portion Size: 1 cup

Stuffed Bell Peppers with Lean Ground Beef and Quinoa

Ingredients:

- 4 bell peppers, halved and seeds removed
- 1 lb lean ground beef
- 1 cup cooked quinoa

- 1 onion, diced

- 2 cloves garlic, minced

- 1 can (15 oz) diced tomatoes

- 1 teaspoon Italian seasoning

- Salt and pepper to taste

- Optional toppings: shredded cheese, chopped parsley

Instructions:

1. Preheat the oven to 375°F (190°C).

2. In a skillet, cook ground beef, onion, and garlic until beef is browned and onion is softened.

3. Stir in cooked quinoa, diced tomatoes, Italian seasoning, salt, and pepper.

4. Arrange bell pepper halves in a baking dish and fill each with the beef and quinoa mixture.

5. Cover the baking dish with foil and bake for 25-30 minutes, or until peppers are tender.

6. Remove from the oven and top with optional toppings before serving.

Nutrition Information:

- Calories: 280

- Protein: 20g
- Carbohydrates: 20g
- Fat: 12g
- Fiber: 4g
- Sugar: 5g
- Portion Size: 2 pepper halves

Veggie Stir-Fry with Tofu and Brown Rice

Ingredients:

- 1 block firm tofu, pressed and cubed
- 2 cups mixed vegetables (such as bell peppers, broccoli, and snap peas)
- 2 tablespoons low-sodium soy sauce
- 1 tablespoon sesame oil
- 2 cloves garlic, minced
- 1 teaspoon ginger, minced
- Cooked brown rice for serving

Instructions:

1. Heat sesame oil in a large skillet over medium heat.

2. Add cubed tofu and cook until golden brown on all sides. Remove from skillet and set aside.

3. In the same skillet, add mixed vegetables, garlic, and ginger. Stir-fry until vegetables are tender-crisp.

4. Return tofu to the skillet and add soy sauce, tossing to combine.

5. Serve hot over cooked brown rice.

Nutrition Information:

- Calories: 320
- Protein: 18g
- Carbohydrates: 40g
- Fat: 10g
- Fiber: 8g
- Sugar: 6g
- Portion Size: 1 cup stir-fry with 1/2 cup brown rice

Grilled Lemon Herb Chicken with Steamed Broccoli

Ingredients:

- 4 boneless, skinless chicken breasts

- 2 tablespoons olive oil

- 2 cloves garlic, minced

- 1 teaspoon lemon zest

- 1 tablespoon fresh lemon juice

- 1 teaspoon dried thyme

- Salt and pepper to taste

- 4 cups broccoli florets

Instructions:

1. In a small bowl, whisk together olive oil, garlic, lemon zest, lemon juice, thyme, salt, and pepper to create a marinade.

2. Place chicken breasts in a shallow dish and pour the marinade over them, ensuring they are evenly coated. Let marinate in the refrigerator for at least 30 minutes.

3. Preheat grill to medium-high heat. Remove chicken from marinade and discard excess marinade.

4. Grill chicken for 6-8 minutes per side, or until fully cooked through and no longer pink in the center.

5. While the chicken is grilling, steam broccoli florets until tender.

6. Serve grilled chicken with steamed broccoli on the
side.

Nutrition Information:

- Calories: 280
- Protein: 30g
- Carbohydrates: 8g
- Fat: 14g
- Fiber: 4g
- Sugar: 2g
- Portion Size: 1 chicken breast with 1 cup broccoli

Spaghetti Squash with Turkey Bolognese Sauce

Ingredients:

- 1 spaghetti squash
- 1 lb lean ground turkey
- 1 onion, diced
- 2 cloves garlic, minced
- 1 can (15 oz) crushed tomatoes
- 1 teaspoon Italian seasoning

- Salt and pepper to taste
- Fresh basil for garnish

Instructions:

1. Preheat the oven to 375°F (190°C). Cut the spaghetti squash in half lengthwise and scoop out the seeds.
2. Place the squash halves, cut side down, on a baking sheet lined with parchment paper. Bake for 30-40 minutes, or until the squash is tender and easily pierced with a fork.
3. While the squash is baking, prepare the turkey bolognese sauce. In a skillet, cook ground turkey, onion, and garlic until turkey is browned and onion is softened.
4. Stir in crushed tomatoes, Italian seasoning, salt, and pepper. Let simmer for 10-15 minutes.
5. Once the spaghetti squash is cooked, use a fork to scrape the flesh into spaghetti-like strands.
6. Serve the spaghetti squash topped with turkey bolognese sauce and garnish with fresh basil.

Nutrition Information:

- Calories: 320
- Protein: 25g
- Carbohydrates: 30g
- Fat: 12g
- Fiber: 8g
- Sugar: 10g
- Portion Size: 1 cup squash with 1 cup sauce

BBQ Chicken Pizza with Whole Wheat Crust

Ingredients:

- 1 whole wheat pizza crust
- 1 cup cooked chicken breast, shredded
- 1/2 cup BBQ sauce
- 1 cup shredded mozzarella cheese
- 1/4 red onion, thinly sliced
- Fresh cilantro for garnish

Instructions:

1. Preheat the oven to 425°F (220°C).

2. Place the whole wheat pizza crust on a baking sheet lined with parchment paper.

3. Spread BBQ sauce evenly over the crust, leaving a small border around the edges.

4. Top with shredded chicken, shredded mozzarella cheese, and thinly sliced red onion.

5. Bake for 12-15 minutes, or until the cheese is melted and bubbly.

6. Remove from the oven and garnish with fresh cilantro before serving.

Nutrition Information:

- Calories: 320
- Protein: 20g
- Carbohydrates: 30g
- Fat: 12g
- Fiber: 4g
- Sugar: 8g
- Portion Size: 1/4 of pizza

Fish Tacos with Mango Salsa

Ingredients:

- 1 lb white fish fillets (such as cod or tilapia)
- 8 small corn tortillas
- 1 mango, diced
- 1/2 red onion, finely chopped
- 1/4 cup fresh cilantro, chopped
- 1 jalapeño, seeded and diced
- Juice of 1 lime
- Salt and pepper to taste
- Optional toppings: shredded cabbage, Greek yogurt, lime wedges

Instructions:

1. Season fish fillets with salt and pepper. Grill or pan-sear until cooked through, about 3-4 minutes per side.
2. Warm corn tortillas on a skillet over medium heat.
3. In a bowl, combine diced mango, chopped red onion, chopped cilantro, diced jalapeño, and lime juice. Season with salt and pepper to taste.

4. Flake cooked fish with a fork and divide among warmed tortillas.

5. Top fish with mango salsa and optional toppings, if desired.

6. Serve immediately.

Nutrition Information:

- Calories: 280
- Protein: 20g
- Carbohydrates: 30g
- Fat: 8g
- Fiber: 6g
- Sugar: 8g
- Portion Size: 2 tacos

Turkey Meatballs with Zucchini Noodles

Ingredients:

- 1 lb lean ground turkey
- 1/4 cup breadcrumbs (whole wheat, if available)
- 1 egg

- 2 cloves garlic, minced

- 1 teaspoon Italian seasoning

- Salt and pepper to taste

- 4 medium zucchini

- Olive oil for cooking

- Marinara sauce for serving

- Fresh basil for garnish

Instructions:

1. In a large mixing bowl, combine ground turkey, breadcrumbs, egg, minced garlic, Italian seasoning, salt, and pepper. Mix until well combined.

2. Roll the turkey mixture into small meatballs, about 1 inch in diameter.

3. Heat olive oil in a skillet over medium heat. Cook meatballs for 8-10 minutes, turning occasionally, until browned on all sides and cooked through.

4. While the meatballs are cooking, spiralize zucchini into noodles using a spiralizer or julienne peeler.

5. In a separate skillet, heat olive oil over medium heat. Add zucchini noodles and sauté for 2-3 minutes, until tender.

6. Serve turkey meatballs over zucchini noodles, topped with marinara sauce and garnished with fresh basil.

Nutrition Information:

- Calories: 280
- Protein: 25g
- Carbohydrates: 15g
- Fat: 12g
- Fiber: 4g
- Sugar: 6g
- Portion Size: 4 meatballs with 1 cup zucchini noodles

Cauliflower Crust Veggie Pizza

Ingredients:

- 1 head cauliflower, riced
- 1 egg
- 1/4 cup grated Parmesan cheese
- 1 teaspoon Italian seasoning
- Salt and pepper to taste
- 1/2 cup marinara sauce

- 1 cup chopped mixed vegetables (such as bell peppers, mushrooms, and onions)
- 1/2 cup shredded mozzarella cheese
- Fresh basil for garnish

Instructions:

1. Preheat the oven to 425°F (220°C). Line a baking sheet with parchment paper.
2. Place riced cauliflower in a microwave-safe bowl and microwave for 5 minutes. Let cool slightly.
3. Transfer cauliflower to a clean kitchen towel and squeeze out excess moisture.
4. In a mixing bowl, combine cauliflower, egg, grated Parmesan cheese, Italian seasoning, salt, and pepper. Mix until a dough forms.
5. Press cauliflower dough onto the prepared baking sheet, forming a pizza crust.
6. Bake crust in the preheated oven for 15-20 minutes, or until golden brown and firm.
7. Spread marinara sauce evenly over the baked crust. Top with chopped vegetables and shredded mozzarella cheese.

8. Return pizza to the oven and bake for an additional 10-12 minutes, or until cheese is melted and bubbly.

9. Garnish with fresh basil before serving.

Nutrition Information:

- Calories: 220
- Protein: 12g
- Carbohydrates: 20g
- Fat: 10g
- Fiber: 6g
- Sugar: 6g
- Portion Size: 1/4 of pizza

Shrimp and Vegetable Skewers with Quinoa

Ingredients:

- 1 lb large shrimp, peeled and deveined
- 2 bell peppers, cut into chunks
- 1 red onion, cut into chunks
- 1 zucchini, sliced
- 1 tablespoon olive oil

- 1 teaspoon garlic powder
- 1 teaspoon paprika
- Salt and pepper to taste
- Cooked quinoa for serving
- Lemon wedges for serving

Instructions:

1. Preheat grill to medium-high heat.
2. In a bowl, toss shrimp, bell peppers, red onion, and zucchini with olive oil, garlic powder, paprika, salt, and pepper until evenly coated.
3. Thread shrimp and vegetables onto skewers, alternating as desired.
4. Grill skewers for 2-3 minutes per side, or until shrimp is pink and vegetables are tender-crisp.
5. Serve skewers over cooked quinoa, with lemon wedges on the side for squeezing over the dish.

Nutrition Information:

- Calories: 280
- Protein: 25g
- Carbohydrates: 20g

- Fat: 10g
- Fiber: 4g
- Sugar: 4g
- Portion Size: 2 skewers with 1/2 cup quinoa

Chicken and Broccoli Alfredo with Whole Wheat Pasta

Ingredients:

- 8 oz whole wheat pasta
- 2 boneless, skinless chicken breasts, cut into bite-sized pieces
- 2 cups broccoli florets
- 1 tablespoon olive oil
- 2 cloves garlic, minced
- 1 cup low-fat milk
- 1/4 cup grated Parmesan cheese
- Salt and pepper to taste
- Fresh parsley for garnish

Instructions:

1. Cook whole wheat pasta according to package instructions. Drain and set aside.
2. In a large skillet, heat olive oil over medium heat. Add chicken pieces and cook until browned and cooked through.
3. Add minced garlic to the skillet and cook for an additional minute.
4. Stir in broccoli florets and cook until tender-crisp.
5. Reduce heat to low and pour in low-fat milk. Stir in grated Parmesan cheese until melted and sauce is creamy.
6. Season with salt and pepper to taste.
7. Add cooked pasta to the skillet and toss until evenly coated with the sauce.
8. Serve hot, garnished with fresh parsley.

Nutrition Information:

- Calories: 380
- Protein: 30g
- Carbohydrates: 40g
- Fat: 12g

- Fiber: 8g
- Sugar: 4g
- Portion Size: 1 cup pasta with chicken and broccoli mixture

Beef and Vegetable Stir-Fry with Cauliflower Rice

Ingredients:

- 1 lb lean beef, thinly sliced
- 2 cups mixed vegetables (such as bell peppers, carrots, and snap peas)
- 1 head cauliflower, riced
- 2 tablespoons low-sodium soy sauce
- 1 tablespoon hoisin sauce
- 1 teaspoon sesame oil
- 2 cloves garlic, minced
- 1 teaspoon ginger, minced
- Salt and pepper to taste
- Green onions for garnish

Instructions:

1. Heat sesame oil in a large skillet or wok over medium-high heat.
2. Add minced garlic and ginger to the skillet and cook for 1 minute.
3. Add sliced beef to the skillet and stir-fry until browned and cooked through.
4. Push the beef to one side of the skillet and add mixed vegetables to the other side. Stir-fry until vegetables are tender-crisp.
5. In a separate skillet, stir-fry cauliflower rice until heated through.
6. In a small bowl, whisk together low-sodium soy sauce and hoisin sauce. Pour over beef and vegetables in the skillet, tossing to coat evenly.
7. Serve beef and vegetable stir-fry over cauliflower rice, garnished with chopped green onions.

Nutrition Information:

- Calories: 320
- Protein: 25g
- Carbohydrates: 20g

- Fat: 14g
- Fiber: 6g
- Sugar: 8g
- Portion Size: 1 cup stir-fry with 1 cup cauliflower rice

Baked Sweet Potato with Black Bean Chili

Ingredients:

- 4 medium sweet potatoes
- 1 can (15 oz) black beans, drained and rinsed
- 1 cup corn kernels
- 1 bell pepper, diced
- 1 onion, diced
- 2 cloves garlic, minced
- 1 can (15 oz) diced tomatoes
- 1 tablespoon chili powder
- 1 teaspoon cumin
- Salt and pepper to taste
- Optional toppings: Greek yogurt, sliced avocado, chopped cilantro

Instructions:

1. Preheat the oven to 400°F (200°C). Pierce sweet potatoes with a fork and place them on a baking sheet lined with parchment paper.
2. Bake sweet potatoes for 45-60 minutes, or until tender.
3. While the sweet potatoes are baking, prepare the black bean chili. In a large pot, sauté diced onion and minced garlic until softened.
4. Add diced bell pepper, black beans, corn kernels, diced tomatoes, chili powder, cumin, salt, and pepper to the pot. Stir to combine.
5. Bring the chili to a simmer and let it cook for 20-25 minutes, stirring occasionally.
6. Once the sweet potatoes are cooked, split them open and fluff the flesh with a fork.
7. Spoon black bean chili over each baked sweet potato and top with optional toppings if desired.

Nutrition Information:
- Calories: 320
- Protein: 10g

- Carbohydrates: 60g

- Fat: 2g

- Fiber: 15g

- Sugar: 12g

- Portion Size: 1 sweet potato with chili topping

Grilled Veggie and Chicken Kabobs with Brown Rice

Ingredients:

- 1 lb boneless, skinless chicken breasts, cut into chunks

- 2 bell peppers, cut into chunks

- 1 zucchini, sliced

- 1 red onion, cut into chunks

- 8 wooden skewers, soaked in water

- 2 tablespoons olive oil

- 2 cloves garlic, minced

- 1 teaspoon dried oregano

- Salt and pepper to taste

- Cooked brown rice for serving

- Lemon wedges for serving

Instructions:

1. Preheat grill to medium-high heat.
2. Thread chicken chunks, bell pepper chunks, zucchini slices, and red onion chunks onto soaked wooden skewers, alternating as desired.
3. In a small bowl, whisk together olive oil, minced garlic, dried oregano, salt, and pepper to create a marinade.
4. Brush marinade over the prepared kabobs.
5. Grill kabobs for 8-10 minutes, turning occasionally, until chicken is cooked through and vegetables are tender.
6. Serve grilled veggie and chicken kabobs over cooked brown rice, with lemon wedges on the side for squeezing over the dish.

Nutrition Information:

- Calories: 350
- Protein: 30g
- Carbohydrates: 30g
- Fat: 12g
- Fiber: 6g

- Sugar: 6g

- Portion Size: 2 skewers with 1/2 cup brown rice

Chapter 5: Snacks and Appetizers

These snacks and appetizers are designed to satisfy cravings while providing essential nutrients and keeping blood sugar levels in check. From crunchy veggie sticks to creamy guacamole, there's something to suit every taste bud and occasion. So, let's dive in and explore these delectable recipes!

Veggie Sticks with Hummus

Ingredients:

- Assorted vegetables (carrots, celery, bell peppers, cucumber)
- Hummus

Instructions:

1. Wash and cut the vegetables into sticks.
2. Serve with a dollop of hummus for dipping.

Nutrition Information (per serving):

- Calories: 100

- Protein: 4g

- Carbohydrates: 12g

- Fat: 5g

- Fiber: 4g

- Sugar: 3g

- Portion Size: 1 cup of vegetables with 2 tablespoons of hummus

Apple Slices with Peanut Butter

Ingredients:

- Apples

- Peanut butter

Instructions:

1. Core and slice the apples.

2. Spread peanut butter on each slice or serve it on the side for dipping.

Nutrition Information (per serving):

- Calories: 150

- Protein: 5g

- Carbohydrates: 18g

- Fat: 8g

- Fiber: 4g

- Sugar: 10g

- Portion Size: 1 medium apple with 2 tablespoons of peanut butter

Yogurt-Covered Frozen Grapes

Ingredients:

- Grapes

- Greek yogurt

Instructions:

1. Wash and dry the grapes.

2. Dip each grape in Greek yogurt until coated.

3. Place the coated grapes on a baking sheet lined with parchment paper.

4. Freeze for at least 2 hours before serving.

Nutrition Information (per serving):

- Calories: 80

- Protein: 3g

- Carbohydrates: 15g

- Fat: 1g
- Fiber: 1g
- Sugar: 10g
- Portion Size: 1 cup of grapes with 2 tablespoons of Greek yogurt coating

Cheese and Whole Grain Crackers

Ingredients:

- Whole grain crackers
- Low-fat cheese slices or cubes

Instructions:

1. Arrange the crackers on a plate.
2. Place cheese slices or cubes on top of each cracker.

Nutrition Information (per serving):

- Calories: 120
- Protein: 6g
- Carbohydrates: 15g
- Fat: 5g
- Fiber: 3g
- Sugar: 2g

- Portion Size: 6 whole grain crackers with 1 ounce of cheese

Popcorn with Parmesan Cheese

Ingredients:

- Popcorn kernels
- Parmesan cheese
- Olive oil (optional)

Instructions:

1. Pop the popcorn kernels using your preferred method.
2. Sprinkle grated Parmesan cheese over the popped popcorn.
3. Drizzle with a small amount of olive oil for extra flavor if desired.

Nutrition Information (per serving):

- Calories: 100
- Protein: 3g
- Carbohydrates: 15g
- Fat: 4g

- Fiber: 3g
- Sugar: 0g
- Portion Size: 3 cups of popcorn with 1 tablespoon of Parmesan cheese

Trail Mix with Nuts and Dried Fruits

Ingredients:

- Assorted nuts (almonds, walnuts, cashews)
- Dried fruits (raisins, cranberries, apricots)

Instructions:

1. Mix the nuts and dried fruits together in a bowl.
2. Portion into individual servings for a convenient snack on the go.

Nutrition Information (per serving):

- Calories: 200
- Protein: 5g
- Carbohydrates: 20g
- Fat: 12g
- Fiber: 4g
- Sugar: 10g

- Portion Size: 1/4 cup of trail mix

Cucumber and Tomato Salad with Balsamic Glaze

Ingredients:

- Cucumbers
- Tomatoes
- Balsamic glaze
- Fresh basil (optional)
- Salt and pepper to taste

Instructions:

1. Slice cucumbers and tomatoes.
2. Arrange on a plate or in a bowl.
3. Drizzle with balsamic glaze.
4. Garnish with fresh basil if desired.
5. Season with salt and pepper to taste.

Nutrition Information (per serving):

- Calories: 50
- Protein: 2g

- Carbohydrates: 10g
- Fat: 1g
- Fiber: 3g
- Sugar: 6g
- Portion Size: 1 cup of salad

Edamame with Sea Salt

Ingredients:

- Edamame (frozen or fresh)
- Sea salt

Instructions:

1. Steam or boil edamame according to package instructions.
2. Drain and sprinkle with sea salt.
3. Serve warm or chilled.

Nutrition Information (per serving):

- Calories: 120
- Protein: 11g
- Carbohydrates: 9g
- Fat: 4g

- Fiber: 5g

- Sugar: 2g

- Portion Size: 1 cup of edamame

Deviled Eggs with Greek Yogurt

Ingredients:

- Hard-boiled eggs

- Greek yogurt

- Dijon mustard

- Paprika

- Salt and pepper to taste

Instructions:

1. Cut hard-boiled eggs in half lengthwise.

2. Remove yolks and place them in a bowl.

3. Mash yolks with Greek yogurt, Dijon mustard, salt, and pepper until smooth.

4. Spoon or pipe the mixture back into the egg whites.

5. Sprinkle with paprika for garnish.

Nutrition Information (per serving):

- Calories: 70

- Protein: 6g
- Carbohydrates: 2g
- Fat: 4g
- Fiber: 0g
- Sugar: 1g
- Portion Size: 2 deviled egg halves

Guacamole with Baked Tortilla Chips

Ingredients:

- Ripe avocados
- Lime juice
- Red onion
- Tomatoes
- Jalapeño (optional)
- Cilantro
- Salt and pepper to taste
- Baked tortilla chips for serving

Instructions:

1. Mash avocados in a bowl.

2. Stir in lime juice, diced red onion, diced tomatoes, diced jalapeño (if using), chopped cilantro, salt, and pepper.
3. Serve with baked tortilla chips.

Nutrition Information (per serving):

- Calories: 150
- Protein: 3g
- Carbohydrates: 10g
- Fat: 12g
- Fiber: 6g
- Sugar: 2g
- Portion Size: 1/4 cup of guacamole with 10 baked tortilla chips

Carrot and Celery Sticks with Ranch Dip

Ingredients:

- Carrots
- Celery
- Ranch dip (store-bought or homemade)

Instructions:

1. Wash and cut carrots and celery into sticks.

2. Serve with ranch dip for dipping.

Nutrition Information (per serving):

- Calories: 80
- Protein: 2g
- Carbohydrates: 10g
- Fat: 4g
- Fiber: 3g
- Sugar: 5g
- Portion Size: 1 cup of vegetables with 2 tablespoons of ranch dip

Greek Yogurt and Berry Popsicles

Ingredients:

- Greek yogurt
- Mixed berries (strawberries, blueberries, raspberries)
- Honey (optional)

Instructions:

1. Mix Greek yogurt with mixed berries in a bowl.

2. Sweeten with honey if desired.

3. Pour mixture into popsicle molds.

4. Insert popsicle sticks and freeze until solid.

Nutrition Information (per serving):

- Calories: 70

- Protein: 5g

- Carbohydrates: 10g

- Fat: 0g

- Fiber: 2g

- Sugar: 7g

- Portion Size: 1 popsicle

Whole Grain Pita Chips with Salsa

Ingredients:

- Whole grain pita bread

- Olive oil

- Salt

- Salsa (store-bought or homemade)

Instructions:

1. Preheat oven to 350°F (175°C).

2. Cut pita bread into triangles.

3. Brush with olive oil and sprinkle with salt.

4. Bake for 10-12 minutes until crispy.

5. Serve with salsa for dipping.

Nutrition Information (per serving):

- Calories: 120
- Protein: 3g
- Carbohydrates: 20g
- Fat: 3g
- Fiber: 4g
- Sugar: 1g
- Portion Size: 6 pita chips with 1/4 cup of salsa

Cottage Cheese with Pineapple Chunks

Ingredients:

- Cottage cheese
- Pineapple chunks (fresh or canned in juice)

Instructions:

1. Spoon cottage cheese into a bowl.

2. Top with pineapple chunks.

Nutrition Information (per serving):

- Calories: 120

- Protein: 13g

- Carbohydrates: 15g

- Fat: 2g

- Fiber: 2g

- Sugar: 12g

- Portion Size: 1/2 cup of cottage cheese with 1/2 cup of pineapple chunks

Baked Sweet Potato Fries with Garlic Aioli

Ingredients:

- Sweet potatoes

- Olive oil

- Garlic powder

- Salt

- Plain Greek yogurt
- Garlic
- Lemon juice

Instructions:

1. Preheat oven to 400°F (200°C).
2. Cut sweet potatoes into fries.
3. Toss with olive oil, garlic powder, and salt.
4. Spread fries in a single layer on a baking sheet.
5. Bake for 25-30 minutes, flipping halfway through.
6. Meanwhile, prepare garlic aioli by mixing Greek yogurt, minced garlic, lemon juice, and salt.
7. Serve sweet potato fries with garlic aioli for dipping.

Nutrition Information (per serving):

- Calories: 150
- Protein: 4g
- Carbohydrates: 25g
- Fat: 4g
- Fiber: 4g
- Sugar: 5g

- Portion Size: 1 cup of sweet potato fries with 2 tablespoons of garlic aioli

Chapter 6: Desserts

In this chapter, we present delectable dessert recipes specially crafted to suit the needs of those with diabetes. From fruity popsicles to decadent chocolate treats, each recipe offers a balance of flavors and textures while providing key nutrition information to help you make informed choices.

Berry and Greek Yogurt Popsicles

Ingredients:

- 1 cup Greek yogurt
- 1 cup mixed berries (strawberries, blueberries, raspberries)
- 2 tablespoons honey or maple syrup (optional)
- Popsicle molds

Instructions:

1. In a blender, combine Greek yogurt, mixed berries, and honey or maple syrup (if using). Blend until smooth.

2. Pour the mixture into popsicle molds, insert sticks, and freeze for at least 4 hours or until solid.

3. Once frozen, remove popsicles from molds and enjoy!

Nutrition Information (per serving):

- Calories: 70
- Protein: 5g
- Carbohydrates: 10g
- Fat: 1g
- Fiber: 2g
- Sugar: 7g
- Portion size: 1 popsicle

Dark Chocolate-Dipped Strawberries

Ingredients:

- 1 cup dark chocolate chips
- 12 large strawberries, washed and dried

Instructions:

1. Melt dark chocolate chips in a microwave-safe bowl in 30-second intervals, stirring between each interval until smooth.

2. Dip each strawberry into the melted chocolate, coating about three-quarters of the berry.

3. Place the dipped strawberries on a parchment-lined baking sheet and refrigerate for 15-20 minutes or until the chocolate sets.

4. Serve and enjoy!

Nutrition Information (per serving, 2 strawberries):

- Calories: 120

- Protein: 2g

- Carbohydrates: 15g

- Fat: 7g

- Fiber: 3g

- Sugar: 10g

- Portion size: 2 strawberries

Baked Apple Crisp with Oats and Cinnamon

Ingredients:

- 4 medium apples, peeled, cored, and sliced

- 1 tablespoon lemon juice

- 1/2 cup old-fashioned oats

- 1/4 cup almond flour

- 2 tablespoons honey or maple syrup

- 1 teaspoon cinnamon

- 2 tablespoons unsalted butter, melted

Instructions:

1. Preheat the oven to 350°F (175°C). Grease a baking dish with non-stick spray.

2. In a large bowl, toss the sliced apples with lemon juice. Transfer the apples to the prepared baking dish.

3. In the same bowl, combine oats, almond flour, honey or maple syrup, cinnamon, and melted butter. Mix until crumbly.

4. Sprinkle the oat mixture evenly over the apples in the baking dish.

5. Bake for 30-35 minutes or until the topping is golden brown and the apples are tender.

6. Serve warm, optionally with a scoop of vanilla Greek yogurt or a drizzle of honey.

Nutrition Information (per serving, 1/6 of recipe):

- Calories: 180
- Protein: 2g
- Carbohydrates: 30g
- Fat: 7g
- Fiber: 5g
- Sugar: 18g
- Portion size: 1/6 of recipe

Frozen Banana Bites with Dark Chocolate

Ingredients:

- 2 ripe bananas, peeled and cut into thick slices
- 1/2 cup dark chocolate chips
- 2 teaspoons coconut oil
- Optional toppings: chopped nuts, shredded coconut, dried fruit

Instructions:

1. Line a baking sheet with parchment paper.

2. Place banana slices on the prepared baking sheet and freeze for 1-2 hours until firm.

3. In a microwave-safe bowl, combine dark chocolate chips and coconut oil. Microwave in 30-second intervals, stirring between each interval until smooth.

4. Using a fork, dip each frozen banana slice into the melted chocolate, coating it halfway. Allow excess chocolate to drip off.

5. Place the chocolate-covered banana slices back onto the parchment-lined baking sheet.

6. Sprinkle with optional toppings if desired.

7. Return the baking sheet to the freezer and freeze until the chocolate is set, about 30 minutes.

8. Once frozen, transfer the banana bites to an airtight container and store in the freezer until ready to serve.

Nutrition Information (per serving, 4 banana bites):

- Calories: 150
- Protein: 2g
- Carbohydrates: 25g
- Fat: 7g
- Fiber: 3g

- Sugar: 14g
- Portion size: 4 banana bites

Lemon Blueberry Parfait with Granola

Ingredients:

- 1 cup Greek yogurt
- 1 tablespoon honey or maple syrup
- Zest of 1 lemon
- 1 cup fresh blueberries
- 1/2 cup granola (choose a low-sugar or homemade variety)

Instructions:

1. In a small bowl, mix Greek yogurt with honey or maple syrup and lemon zest until well combined.
2. In serving glasses or bowls, layer the Greek yogurt mixture, fresh blueberries, and granola.
3. Repeat the layers until the glasses are filled, ending with a sprinkle of granola on top.
4. Serve immediately or refrigerate until ready to enjoy.

Nutrition Information (per serving):

- Calories: 220
- Protein: 10g
- Carbohydrates: 35g
- Fat: 5g
- Fiber: 4g
- Sugar: 20g
- Portion size: 1 serving

Chia Seed Pudding with Mixed Berries

Ingredients:

- 1/4 cup chia seeds
- 1 cup unsweetened almond milk
- 1 tablespoon honey or maple syrup
- 1/2 teaspoon vanilla extract
- 1 cup mixed berries (strawberries, blueberries, raspberries)

Instructions:

1. In a mixing bowl, whisk together chia seeds, almond milk, honey or maple syrup, and vanilla extract.

2. Let the mixture sit for 5 minutes, then whisk again to prevent clumping.

3. Cover the bowl and refrigerate for at least 2 hours or overnight, allowing the chia seeds to thicken and absorb the liquid.

4. Before serving, stir the chia seed pudding to loosen it up and divide it into serving bowls.

5. Top with mixed berries and serve chilled.

Nutrition Information (per serving):

- Calories: 180
- Protein: 5g
- Carbohydrates: 25g
- Fat: 8g
- Fiber: 9g
- Sugar: 12g
- Portion size: 1 serving

Pumpkin Pie Energy Bites

Ingredients:

- 1 cup rolled oats
- 1/2 cup pumpkin puree
- 1/4 cup almond butter
- 2 tablespoons honey or maple syrup
- 1 teaspoon pumpkin pie spice
- 1/4 cup chopped pecans or walnuts (optional)

Instructions:

1. In a large mixing bowl, combine rolled oats, pumpkin puree, almond butter, honey or maple syrup, and pumpkin pie spice. Mix until well combined.
2. If desired, fold in chopped pecans or walnuts for added crunch and flavor.
3. Roll the mixture into bite-sized balls using your hands.
4. Place the energy bites on a parchment-lined baking sheet and refrigerate for at least 30 minutes to firm up.

5. Once firm, transfer the energy bites to an airtight container and store in the refrigerator until ready to enjoy.

Nutrition Information (per serving, 2 energy bites):

- Calories: 120
- Protein: 3g
- Carbohydrates: 15g
- Fat: 6g
- Fiber: 2g
- Sugar: 6g
- Portion size: 2 energy bites

Greek Yogurt Bark with Berries and Nuts

Ingredients:

- 2 cups Greek yogurt
- 2 tablespoons honey or maple syrup
- 1/2 cup mixed berries (strawberries, blueberries, raspberries)
- 1/4 cup chopped nuts (almonds, walnuts, pecans)

- Optional toppings: shredded coconut, dark chocolate chips

Instructions:

1. Line a baking sheet with parchment paper.
2. In a mixing bowl, combine Greek yogurt and honey or maple syrup until smooth.
3. Spread the Greek yogurt mixture evenly onto the prepared baking sheet, about 1/4-inch thick.
4. Sprinkle mixed berries, chopped nuts, and any other desired toppings over the yogurt layer.
5. Place the baking sheet in the freezer and freeze for 2-3 hours or until firm.
6. Once frozen, break the yogurt bark into pieces and serve immediately, or transfer to an airtight container and store in the freezer for later enjoyment.

Nutrition Information (per serving, 1/8 of recipe):

- Calories: 90
- Protein: 6g
- Carbohydrates: 10g
- Fat: 4g

- Fiber: 1g
- Sugar: 7g
- Portion size: 1/8 of recipe

Mango Sorbet with Lime Zest

Ingredients:

- 2 cups frozen mango chunks
- 1/4 cup water
- Zest of 1 lime
- Optional sweetener: honey or maple syrup (to taste)

Instructions:

1. In a blender or food processor, combine frozen mango chunks, water, and lime zest.
2. Blend until smooth, adding sweetener if desired for extra sweetness.
3. Transfer the mixture to a shallow dish and spread it out evenly.
4. Place the dish in the freezer and freeze for at least 4 hours or until firm.
5. Before serving, let the sorbet sit at room temperature for a few minutes to soften slightly.

6. Scoop the mango sorbet into bowls or cones and enjoy!

Nutrition Information (per serving):

- Calories: 80
- Protein: 1g
- Carbohydrates: 20g
- Fat: 0g
- Fiber: 2g
- Sugar: 18g
- Portion size: 1 serving

Almond Flour Chocolate Chip Cookies

Ingredients:

- 2 cups almond flour
- 1/4 cup coconut oil, melted
- 1/4 cup honey or maple syrup
- 1 teaspoon vanilla extract
- 1/2 teaspoon baking soda
- 1/4 teaspoon salt

- 1/2 cup dark chocolate chips

Instructions:

1. Preheat the oven to 350°F (175°C). Line a baking sheet with parchment paper.

2. In a large mixing bowl, combine almond flour, melted coconut oil, honey or maple syrup, vanilla extract, baking soda, and salt. Mix until well combined.

3. Fold in the dark chocolate chips until evenly distributed throughout the dough.

4. Scoop tablespoon-sized portions of dough and roll them into balls. Place the balls on the prepared baking sheet and flatten slightly with the palm of your hand.

5. Bake in the preheated oven for 10-12 minutes, or until the edges are golden brown.

6. Remove from the oven and let the cookies cool on the baking sheet for 5 minutes before transferring them to a wire rack to cool completely.

Nutrition Information (per serving, 1 cookie):

- Calories: 120
- Protein: 3g
- Carbohydrates: 10g
- Fat: 9g
- Fiber: 2g
- Sugar: 6g
- Portion size: 1 cookie

Strawberry Banana Smoothie Bowl with Granola

Ingredients:

- 1 ripe banana, sliced and frozen
- 1 cup frozen strawberries
- 1/2 cup Greek yogurt
- 1/4 cup almond milk
- Toppings: granola, fresh strawberries, sliced banana, shredded coconut

Instructions:

1. In a blender, combine frozen banana slices, frozen strawberries, Greek yogurt, and almond milk. Blend until smooth and creamy.

2. Pour the smoothie into a bowl and top with granola, fresh strawberries, sliced banana, and shredded coconut.

3. Serve immediately and enjoy with a spoon!

Nutrition Information (per serving):

- Calories: 200
- Protein: 8g
- Carbohydrates: 35g
- Fat: 5g
- Fiber: 6g
- Sugar: 18g
- Portion size: 1 serving

Coconut Macaroons with Dark Chocolate Drizzle

Ingredients:

- 3 cups shredded coconut
- 3/4 cup sweetened condensed milk
- 1 teaspoon vanilla extract
- 2 large egg whites
- Pinch of salt
- 1/2 cup dark chocolate chips, melted

Instructions:

1. Preheat the oven to 325°F (160°C). Line a baking sheet with parchment paper.
2. In a large mixing bowl, combine shredded coconut, sweetened condensed milk, and vanilla extract. Mix until well combined.
3. In a separate bowl, beat egg whites with a pinch of salt until stiff peaks form.
4. Gently fold the beaten egg whites into the coconut mixture until evenly incorporated.

5. Drop tablespoon-sized portions of the mixture onto
    the prepared baking sheet, spacing them about 1 inch
    apart.
6. Bake in the preheated oven for 20-25 minutes or until
    the macaroons are golden brown around the edges.
7. Remove from the oven and let the macaroons cool
    completely on the baking sheet.
8. Once cooled, drizzle melted dark chocolate over the
    macaroons using a fork or spoon.
9. Let the chocolate set before serving.

Nutrition Information (per serving, 2 macaroons):

- Calories: 150
- Protein: 2g
- Carbohydrates: 15g
- Fat: 10g
- Fiber: 2g
- Sugar: 12g
- Portion size: 2 macaroons

Frozen Yogurt Fruit Bark

Ingredients:

- 2 cups plain Greek yogurt
- 2 tablespoons honey or maple syrup
- 1 teaspoon vanilla extract
- 1 cup mixed fresh fruit (such as berries, sliced kiwi, and mango)
- 1/4 cup granola
- Optional toppings: shredded coconut, dark chocolate chips

Instructions:

1. Line a baking sheet with parchment paper.
2. In a mixing bowl, combine Greek yogurt, honey or maple syrup, and vanilla extract. Stir until smooth and well combined.
3. Spread the Greek yogurt mixture evenly onto the prepared baking sheet, about 1/4-inch thick.
4. Arrange mixed fresh fruit over the yogurt layer, pressing gently to adhere.
5. Sprinkle granola and any optional toppings over the fruit layer.

6. Place the baking sheet in the freezer and freeze for 2-3 hours or until firm.

7. Once frozen, break the yogurt bark into pieces and serve immediately, or transfer to an airtight container and store in the freezer for later enjoyment.

Nutrition Information (per serving, 1/8 of recipe):

- Calories: 90
- Protein: 6g
- Carbohydrates: 15g
- Fat: 1g
- Fiber: 2g
- Sugar: 10g
- Portion size: 1/8 of recipe

Peanut Butter Banana Bites

Ingredients:

- 2 bananas, peeled and sliced into rounds
- 2 tablespoons peanut butter (or any nut or seed butter)
- Optional toppings: chopped nuts, dark chocolate chips, shredded coconut

Instructions:

1. Spread peanut butter onto one side of each banana slice.

2. Place another banana slice on top to form a "sandwich."

3. If desired, roll the edges of the banana sandwiches in chopped nuts, dark chocolate chips, or shredded coconut to coat.

4. Arrange the banana bites on a plate or baking sheet lined with parchment paper.

5. Place the plate or baking sheet in the freezer and freeze for 1-2 hours or until firm.

6. Once frozen, transfer the banana bites to an airtight container and store in the freezer until ready to serve.

Nutrition Information (per serving, 4 banana bites):

- Calories: 150
- Protein: 4g
- Carbohydrates: 20g
- Fat: 7g
- Fiber: 3g
- Sugar: 12g

- Portion size: 4 banana bites

Avocado Chocolate Mousse

Ingredients:

- 2 ripe avocados, peeled and pitted
- 1/4 cup unsweetened cocoa powder
- 1/4 cup honey or maple syrup
- 1 teaspoon vanilla extract
- Pinch of salt
- Optional toppings: whipped cream, shaved dark chocolate, fresh berries

Instructions:

1. In a food processor or blender, combine ripe avocados, cocoa powder, honey or maple syrup, vanilla extract, and a pinch of salt.
2. Blend until smooth and creamy, scraping down the sides of the bowl as needed.
3. Taste the mousse and adjust sweetness if necessary by adding more honey or maple syrup.
4. Transfer the chocolate avocado mousse to serving bowls or glasses.

5. Refrigerate for at least 30 minutes to chill and set.

6. Before serving, top with whipped cream, shaved dark chocolate, and fresh berries if desired.

Nutrition Information (per serving, 1/4 of recipe):

- Calories: 180
- Protein: 3g
- Carbohydrates: 20g
- Fat: 12g
- Fiber: 6g
- Sugar: 12g
- Portion size: 1/4 of recipe

Chapter 7: Smoothies

In this chapter, we present unique smoothie recipes designed to tantalize your taste buds while supporting your health goals. Each recipe is carefully crafted to include diabetic-friendly ingredients and comes with detailed instructions for preparation.

Green Monster Smoothie with Spinach and Banana

Ingredients:

- 1 ripe banana
- 1 cup fresh spinach leaves
- ½ cup unsweetened almond milk
- ½ cup plain Greek yogurt
- 1 tablespoon honey (optional)
- Ice cubes (optional)

Instructions:

1. Peel the banana and break it into chunks.

2. In a blender, combine the banana chunks, spinach leaves, almond milk, Greek yogurt, and honey (if using).

3. Blend until smooth and creamy, adding ice cubes if desired for a colder consistency.

4. Pour into glasses and serve immediately.

Nutrition Information:

- Calories: 150
- Protein: 8g
- Carbohydrates: 28g
- Fat: 2g
- Fiber: 3g
- Sugar: 18g
- Portion Size: 1 serving

Berry Blast Smoothie with Greek Yogurt

Ingredients:

- 1 cup mixed berries (strawberries, blueberries, raspberries)

- ½ cup plain Greek yogurt

- ½ cup unsweetened almond milk

- 1 tablespoon honey (optional)

- Ice cubes (optional)

Instructions:

1. Rinse the mixed berries and remove any stems.

2. In a blender, combine the mixed berries, Greek yogurt, almond milk, and honey (if using).

3. Blend until smooth and creamy, adding ice cubes if desired.

4. Pour into glasses and serve immediately.

Nutrition Information:

- Calories: 120

- Protein: 6g

- Carbohydrates: 20g

- Fat: 2g

- Fiber: 4g

- Sugar: 14g

- Portion Size: 1 serving

Tropical Paradise Smoothie with Pineapple and Mango

Ingredients:

- 1 cup diced pineapple
- 1 cup diced mango
- ½ cup coconut milk
- ½ cup unsweetened almond milk
- 1 tablespoon lime juice
- Ice cubes (optional)

Instructions:

1. In a blender, combine the diced pineapple, mango, coconut milk, almond milk, and lime juice.
2. Blend until smooth and creamy, adding ice cubes if desired for a colder texture.
3. Pour into glasses and serve immediately.

Nutrition Information:

- Calories: 180
- Protein: 2g
- Carbohydrates: 35g
- Fat: 5g

- Fiber: 4g

- Sugar: 28g

- Portion Size: 1 serving

Chocolate Peanut Butter Protein Smoothie

Ingredients:

- 1 ripe banana

- 2 tablespoons unsweetened cocoa powder

- 2 tablespoons natural peanut butter

- 1 cup unsweetened almond milk

- ½ cup plain Greek yogurt

- Ice cubes (optional)

Instructions:

1. Peel the banana and break it into chunks.

2. In a blender, combine the banana chunks, cocoa powder, peanut butter, almond milk, and Greek yogurt.

3. Blend until smooth and creamy, adding ice cubes if desired.

4. Pour into glasses and serve immediately.

Nutrition Information:

- Calories: 280
- Protein: 15g
- Carbohydrates: 30g
- Fat: 12g
- Fiber: 6g
- Sugar: 14g
- Portion Size: 1 serving

Kale and Apple Smoothie with Almond Milk

Ingredients:

- 1 cup chopped kale leaves
- 1 medium apple, cored and chopped
- ½ cup unsweetened almond milk
- ½ cup plain Greek yogurt
- 1 tablespoon honey (optional)
- Ice cubes (optional)

Instructions:

1. In a blender, combine the chopped kale leaves, chopped apple, almond milk, Greek yogurt, and honey (if using).
2. Blend until smooth and creamy, adding ice cubes if desired for a colder consistency.
3. Pour into glasses and serve immediately.

Nutrition Information:

- Calories: 140
- Protein: 8g
- Carbohydrates: 25g
- Fat: 2g
- Fiber: 5g
- Sugar: 16g
- Portion Size: 1 serving

Mango Tango Smoothie with Coconut Milk

Ingredients:

- 1 cup diced mango

- ½ cup coconut milk
- ½ cup plain Greek yogurt
- 1 tablespoon lime juice
- Ice cubes (optional)

Instructions:

1. In a blender, combine the diced mango, coconut milk, Greek yogurt, and lime juice.
2. Blend until smooth and creamy, adding ice cubes if desired for a colder texture.
3. Pour into glasses and serve immediately.

Nutrition Information:

- Calories: 200
- Protein: 6g
- Carbohydrates: 30g
- Fat: 8g
- Fiber: 3g
- Sugar: 25g
- Portion Size: 1 serving

Peachy Keen Smoothie with Greek Yogurt

Ingredients:

- 1 cup sliced peaches (fresh or frozen)
- ½ cup plain Greek yogurt
- ½ cup unsweetened almond milk
- 1 tablespoon honey (optional)
- Ice cubes (optional)

Instructions:

1. In a blender, combine the sliced peaches, Greek yogurt, almond milk, and honey (if using).
2. Blend until smooth and creamy, adding ice cubes if desired.
3. Pour into glasses and serve immediately.

Nutrition Information:

- Calories: 140
- Protein: 8g
- Carbohydrates: 25g
- Fat: 2g
- Fiber: 3g

- Sugar: 20g
- Portion Size: 1 serving

Strawberry Banana Protein Smoothie with Spinach

Ingredients:

- 1 ripe banana
- 1 cup sliced strawberries
- 1 cup fresh spinach leaves
- ½ cup unsweetened almond milk
- ½ cup plain Greek yogurt
- Ice cubes (optional)

Instructions:

1. Peel the banana and break it into chunks.
2. In a blender, combine the banana chunks, sliced strawberries, spinach leaves, almond milk, and Greek yogurt.
3. Blend until smooth and creamy, adding ice cubes if desired.
4. Pour into glasses and serve immediately.

Nutrition Information:

- Calories: 160
- Protein: 10g
- Carbohydrates: 28g
- Fat: 2g
- Fiber: 6g
- Sugar: 16g
- Portion Size: 1 serving

Blueberry Almond Butter Smoothie

Ingredients:

- 1 cup blueberries (fresh or frozen)
- 2 tablespoons almond butter
- ½ cup unsweetened almond milk
- ½ cup plain Greek yogurt
- 1 tablespoon honey (optional)
- Ice cubes (optional)

Instructions:

1. In a blender, combine the blueberries, almond butter, almond milk, Greek yogurt, and honey (if using).

2. Blend until smooth and creamy, adding ice cubes if desired.

3. Pour into glasses and serve immediately.

Nutrition Information:

- Calories: 220
- Protein: 8g
- Carbohydrates: 25g
- Fat: 12g
- Fiber: 5g
- Sugar: 18g
- Portion Size: 1 serving

Avocado Spinach Smoothie with Kiwi

Ingredients:

- 1 ripe avocado, peeled and pitted
- 1 kiwi, peeled and chopped
- 1 cup fresh spinach leaves
- ½ cup unsweetened almond milk
- ½ cup plain Greek yogurt

- Ice cubes (optional)

Instructions:

1. In a blender, combine the ripe avocado, chopped kiwi, spinach leaves, almond milk, and Greek yogurt.
2. Blend until smooth and creamy, adding ice cubes if desired.
3. Pour into glasses and serve immediately.

Nutrition Information:

- Calories: 230
- Protein: 10g
- Carbohydrates: 20g
- Fat: 14g
- Fiber: 9g
- Sugar: 9g
- Portion Size: 1 serving

Carrot Cake Smoothie with Cinnamon

Ingredients:

- 1 cup chopped carrots
- 1 ripe banana
- ½ cup unsweetened almond milk
- ½ cup plain Greek yogurt
- 1 tablespoon maple syrup
- ½ teaspoon ground cinnamon
- Ice cubes (optional)

Instructions:

1. In a blender, combine the chopped carrots, banana, almond milk, Greek yogurt, maple syrup, and ground cinnamon.
2. Blend until smooth and creamy, adding ice cubes if desired.
3. Pour into glasses and serve immediately.

Nutrition Information:

- Calories: 170
- Protein: 8g

- Carbohydrates: 30g
- Fat: 2g
- Fiber: 5g
- Sugar: 18g
- Portion Size: 1 serving

Piña Colada Smoothie with Coconut Water

Ingredients:

- 1 cup diced pineapple
- ½ cup diced mango
- ½ cup coconut water
- ½ cup plain Greek yogurt
- 1 tablespoon shredded coconut
- Ice cubes (optional)

Instructions:

1. In a blender, combine the diced pineapple, diced mango, coconut water, Greek yogurt, and shredded coconut.

2. Blend until smooth and creamy, adding ice cubes if desired.

3. Pour into glasses and serve immediately.

Nutrition Information:

- Calories: 160
- Protein: 8g
- Carbohydrates: 30g
- Fat: 2g
- Fiber: 3g
- Sugar: 20g
- Portion Size: 1 serving

Beetroot Berry Smoothie with Orange Juice

Ingredients:

- 1 small beetroot, peeled and chopped
- 1 cup mixed berries (strawberries, raspberries, blueberries)
- ½ cup orange juice
- ½ cup plain Greek yogurt

- 1 tablespoon honey (optional)
- Ice cubes (optional)

Instructions:

1. In a blender, combine the chopped beetroot, mixed berries, orange juice, Greek yogurt, and honey (if using).
2. Blend until smooth and creamy, adding ice cubes if desired.
3. Pour into glasses and serve immediately.

Nutrition Information:

- Calories: 160
- Protein: 8g
- Carbohydrates: 30g
- Fat: 2g
- Fiber: 5g
- Sugar: 22g
- Portion Size: 1 serving

Cucumber Mint Smoothie with Honeydew Melon

Ingredients:

- 1 cup diced honeydew melon
- ½ cucumber, peeled and chopped
- 1 tablespoon fresh mint leaves
- ½ cup coconut water
- ½ cup plain Greek yogurt
- 1 tablespoon lime juice
- Ice cubes (optional)

Instructions:

1. In a blender, combine the diced honeydew melon, chopped cucumber, mint leaves, coconut water, Greek yogurt, and lime juice.
2. Blend until smooth and creamy, adding ice cubes if desired.
3. Pour into glasses and serve immediately.

Nutrition Information:

- Calories: 140
- Protein: 8g

- Carbohydrates: 25g
- Fat: 2g
- Fiber: 3g
- Sugar: 18g
- Portion Size: 1 serving

Cherry Vanilla Smoothie with Almond Milk

Ingredients:

- 1 cup pitted cherries (fresh or frozen)
- ½ teaspoon vanilla extract
- ½ cup unsweetened almond milk
- ½ cup plain Greek yogurt
- 1 tablespoon honey (optional)
- Ice cubes (optional)

Instructions:

1. In a blender, combine the pitted cherries, vanilla extract, almond milk, Greek yogurt, and honey (if using).

2. Blend until smooth and creamy, adding ice cubes if desired.

3. Pour into glasses and serve immediately.

Nutrition Information:

- Calories: 160
- Protein: 8g
- Carbohydrates: 25g
- Fat: 2g
- Fiber: 3g
- Sugar: 20g
- Portion Size: 1 serving

CONCLUSION

"Kid-Friendly Recipes for Type 2 Diabetes" serves as a beacon of hope and practical guidance for families navigating the complexities of managing diabetes while ensuring their children enjoy delicious, nutritious meals. Through the careful curation of diverse recipes spanning breakfast, lunch, dinner, snacks, desserts, and smoothies, this book empowers caregivers with the tools to foster healthier eating habits without sacrificing flavor or variety.

Beyond the culinary realm, this book embodies a journey of education and empowerment. It illuminates the path toward understanding the nuances of type 2 diabetes in children and the critical role that diet plays in its management. By presenting a 30-day meal plan and a plethora of recipes carefully crafted to meet the nutritional needs of young ones with diabetes, it instills confidence and reassurance in caregivers, knowing they have the resources to support their child's health journey.

However, this book is more than just a collection of recipes. It's a testament to resilience, adaptability, and the power of community. It encourages families to come together around the dinner table, fostering bonds and shared experiences while nourishing both body and soul. It reminds us that with knowledge, creativity, and a dash of culinary magic, we can transform everyday meals into vibrant celebrations of health and wellness.

As we bid farewell to these pages, let us carry forward the lessons learned and the flavors savored, embracing a future filled with delicious possibilities and a renewed commitment to the well-being of our loved ones. May this book serve as a trusted companion on your journey toward a healthier, happier life, one bite at a time.

www.ingramcontent.com/pod-product-compliance
Lightning Source LLC
Chambersburg PA
CBHW061638250726
48659CB00004B/1274